INTO THE WORLD OF MEN

INTO THE WORLD OF MEN

David Raffeld

Illustration by Julio Granda

ADASTRA PRESS
Easthampton, Massachusetts

First Edition

ISBN 0-938566-74-1 cloth
ISBN 0-938566-75-X paper

Adastra Press
101 Strong Street
Easthampton, Massachusetts 01027

Dedicated to the Memory
of my Parents
Eleanor and Leonard Raffeld

Contents

Into the World of Men

WITH my lunch box holding
the last quartered apple of the moon
cushioned above the Dostoevsky short stories
buried in the bottom dark, I entered the world of men
at 5AM riding the South Chicago train
from Hyde Park to the Little Calumet River stop.
It was my first job so far from home.
Carpenter's apprentice, I was illegal at fifteen
thanks to an Uncle with clout
in the gargoyled world of graft
in the city of How Things Got Done.
At a USA housing project for the poor,
the air borne fat on the sweet smell of potatoes
fried in oil at the Jays potato chip factory
down the road, a special waffled hammer
nailed my days of sheet rock shut.
I left seven impressions from the seven nails
I drove in every line of every half sheet
on the wall, seven dimpled circles in a city
Dante would never strut, and with my metal snippers
cut right angles in the eight foot perforated aluminum
bead to cover rough edges and imperfect corners.

At noon, boss Pete, the former World Rodeo Champ,
inspected my work. Barely able to stand
on his washed up wish bone legs
bucked from one too many broncs,

with only a silver buckle and a shiny new pickup
to show for all his truck I'd pass
while he'd complain about the men
working below: The "wet backs" in the basement;
Leonardo, Juan, Pablo, and Jorge,
who worked from six to six for a buck an hour,
who folded their dollars like tortillas
filled with dreams of bringing their families
one by one to Chicago. In five & dime gym shoes,
clotheslines for belts holding their spackled
pants up, sweat steaming off their bodies
like hot tamales from the lunch wagon bin,
they swore by the holy virgin at their lousy wages
while pissing and shitting in the corners
of the very basements we worked salvaging
sheetrock scraps to piecemeal walls.
And when Pete complained about the smell
and told them to use the sanolets, Leonardo said,
"Boss for extra buck an hour we go outside."
What did I know about days
government inspectors would show
and all the illegals on the site turned
from sheetrock into water and disappeared.
I was the one still wet behind the ears.

But I learned to keep my mouth shut
tight as the corners I made.
Especially around the Tennessee studs

whose 'chawed' teeth were wedged open
from firing dry wall nails into the 'rock.'
Two Herculean rednecks at a dollar a sheet
could put up 140 sheets a day.
These same men who guzzled Schlitz
gawked at stroke books while they ate,
couldn't or wouldn't joke about that summer after-
noon
a mile from where we worked
when Richard Speck's tattoo,
'born to raise hell', rose in the national news
like the Chicago walls we built
so hastily and cheaply erect.

So Easy

It should be so easy
walking into my room
the leaves doing the work:
raking the alphabet; clearing
old ground for the new litter
of maples, oaks, marigolds;
stuffing every bit and thistle
of Autumn into my hat—
antler and cocoon dust,
chrysalis shadow, woody tooth of a star
broken off the bridge
of God's poor fumbling mouth.

It should be so easy,
the old glutton of school days
force feeding snow down my throat,
rage sandwiched between frozen twigs
and mold. My tongue an ice-scabbed
Chicago city street cracked from weeds
breaking through my ancestry: Indiana chicken farmer,
Sephardi rag picker Jew, whose sand blistered blood
rings with eighth grade fists at the recess bell:
Whose sister? KikeSpicCommieBastardWhore!

It should be so easy,
riding the Hard Luck Line,
not having to pay for the bumps

on the way. *Fly on the wings of my grave,*
the good book says and splits my spine
as it whistles for the jackknife wind to bind
my fate to city boy life:

I bus my dreams;
my woman is a perfect spoon ladling
all the silver of the moon into a one night stand.
She leans on my shoulder as the EL
leans into the curve. She leads me
into the four winds that ride
the burning rail of her room
where I'm free to lose everything
I never had no how.

It should be so easy—
As if Michelangelo never ran out of stone,
or the stone in Michelangelo
walked back into the mountain
it was carved from, saying, "Nothing
is immortal. Bronze the shape of the wind.
Catch a fly in the cup of your hand
missing its fingers."

It should be so easy.
The moon a night cap:
A pond drinking up the mirror

of starlight fish flying through a parable
of unbroken days.
Not one splash.
Only measured silver drops.

Spanky's

And they were there
in an East Gary whorehouse
a dozen or so boys
making a Chevy caravan of Friday nights
Spanky's they would say
and a white Cadillac born inside a jazz riff
Spanky's and the poker table chips
would fall like the stars and stripes
off the little white boy souls of South Chicago
who gave away their money and spilled their seed

Spanky's and the nights along the Calumet humid
and the stars would cross themselves and not bleed
for the little white souls at Spanky's
as they jumped out their cars at the state line
buying up fireworks
carbon chips that burst
into black snakes lit on city concrete
that turned into ash on the Fourth
And later around the table the steel men
who made ball bearings at the mill
and the black ladies in the parlor would roar
about showin them sorry white boys where it should
go

Listen

to them breathing
the ash of their families
'die Juden' working the air
words like scraps of black cloth
rent before spoken

'die Kinder'
naked as winter kindling
shivering
clawing concrete floor

the broken declensions of a Roman noun
to Jesus son father and holy corpse
give thanks for the food
for hunger that's fed
by potatoes born
of the oven's daily flow
bread of the ash
of your family's blood and bone

the muzzle on your neck Isaac
you, who stand between 'Moses Of The No Law'
and 'Elijah Of The No God'
as Aaron loses his sons and daughters
to the wheel of fire
Sarah Rebecca Rachel Leah Ruth

Daniel   where is your horn
Give us a song
something to trumpet
a name

Chicken Soup

It took an hour to get there,
an hour back and we had to be home
before Friday sundown was why my grandmother
drove 75 in a 30 zone from the southeast
to the northwest side of Chicago
to get our three kosher chickens.
We drove through the long bearded streets,
weeping willow vines that were only a little longer
than the sideburns of the Hasids we passed
hurrying in preparation for the Sabbath.
When we got to the garage behind the Rabbi's house
I heard chicken squawks and smelled ammonia.

Waiting inside, customers ordered in Yiddish
and in Yiddish the Reb said the prayer
as he grabbed the chicken by its feet,
turned it upside down and slit its throat.
As my grandmother handed the Reb's helper
a little extra for plucking, the garage floor sprouted
more white feathers blotched with the blood that flowed.
Wrapped up in day old news, we carried
our dead chickens home.

My brother liked the feet,
my father the white meat, my sister the dark,
but always there was the feather my grandmother planted
in my grandfather's soup so she could complain

about the chicken plucking, so that my grandfather,
Solomon, could say, "It's alright, Ester, the feather
is for the chicken so he shouldn't forget
what a good soup."

Red Is Dead Warhol, Too

Tarco Terry and me
would sneak down the basement stairs
like spies through the canvas 'iron curtain'
into the room where Tarco's
dad kept the ham radio set.
We listened to Radio Free Europe
surrounded by the maps his father kept:
Little red flags with the hammer and sickle
and pins sticking out along the coastal shores
where the 'Commies' would attack.
This was 1957. We were both eight,
and outside the Palmer House Hotel
in downtown Chicago protesters waved
signs, like "I'd Rather Be Dead Than Red",
while we listened to the broadcast
that armed our fears, and Mr. Terry built
the only fall out shelter on our block:
A ten by ten room, three feet of brick
thick enough to take a nuclear shock.
Tarco's dad stacked supplies:
juices, surplus rations, portable stove,
potable water, blankets, candles, medicines.
Indeed he was set to survive
with his five great books, and manuals
for starting the world up again
when he had a heart attack
carrying a case of Campbell's Tomato Soup
down the stairs
and died.

Tea Ceremony

Mid afternoon, July 1991:
Four of us sit on Adirondacks surrounded
by Evergreen, Juniper and Scotch Pine,
Robin bird song as we stretch our legs
after lunch and the talk turns to Vietnam:
Some of the better books about the war
(although only two of us served)
when Willy takes off his sunglasses,
says, "ours was the unit the brass hand picked
with the best sharp shooters in all of Nam.
You see, the North Vietnamese
believed they couldn't get into heaven
without their eyes. So after we killed em
we gouged them out."

Willy puts his sunglasses back on.
I fill glasses with ice.
Listen to it jingle.
Ask if anyone wants some tea.

The Model

He told me
how just after hearing
of his father's death
his fingers chilled
the blade that cut through layers
of muscle, tendon, tissue.
Perfectly exposed
his dissection of the hand
became the medical school model.

Nirvana

A few Sundays a year Edith Levitan
and my mother ate strudel upstairs
while Eugene, her palsied son, and I
played furiously in the basement.
With a single chain light bulb for light,
a rattling old washing machine for a beat,
Gene waved his arms prolonging
the syllables of my name until I woke
to his awakening. Juggler, I'd toss red, green,
yellow, blue rubber balls that bounced off our heads
like chaos colliding in a rainbow. Then I'd fall
to the ground, bark, growl. Leopard, I'd leap
onto a ratty chair, yell like a banshee
calling out the moon.

Gene would laugh and laugh
his head rollicking back and forth like a bean bag,
the saliva foaming out the corner of his mouth like
holy bilge
until he could laugh no more and his head tilted
to one side, a paperweight keeping everything
but the spastic arms down.
And when he left, before his mother
carried him in his wheel chair up the stairs,
Eugene extended the 'steady' hand
and we'd shake all over Time.
Bless his crooked arms and hands
for the audience he gave me
I would never have again.

Dishrag Dog

Dishrag dog got sorrow in her bones.
Comes to class with a welt on her arm.
Watchdad dog tattoo his charm
on all her limbs cause he thinks it's his right
break the bread of his daughter all through the
night.
Dishrag does her math by counting bruises
multiplied by the square root of what she loses,
divides it by the angle
of the hypotenuse of fear.
Her solution: bronze the tears.
Dishrag dog, ten years old,
beats the sorrow on her sister
with her dog food bowl.

Shoes

"Somebody give me a shoehorn,"
the old man says leaning on a maple tree,
the leaves' golden loaves turning in the sun.
"I have these shoes. Yesterday they fit.
I took them off only a second ago.
Look how my feet swell. They're so bloated
my veins hug the shoreline of unkneaded flesh,
and how around the cold blue rivers of my blood
the lining of my capillary walls crumble like chalk
not even good for writing."

"If only I had a shoehorn..."
The noon sun strikes the clock inside the tree
and the bark rings out, winds itself up
from the roots down and no one sees.
Like the old man, the tree thinks,
if it could think. "Please," the old man says again.
But this please is more music than regret.

The afternoon crawls like a spider
inching down the sun's latticed web.
The old man kneels,
gathers leaves to make his pillow
harvest sleep. Laying down he sighs.
He is glad there is no shoehorn.
If there were he would have to try

and if he succeeded he would have to rise.
Already he can hear his breath climbing,
first out of his mouth, then his heart.
He looks down but cannot see
the white moth fluttering
above the black ridges of his shoes.

Newton's Worm

Not long
before his apple falls
the clapboard wind slaps the tree
its gust rocks the branches
as sun polished light
drizzles through the leaves.
Below, cozy in his moldy cove
of debris, worm recalls his loft,
the catacombs of apples
he ate into sky.
Referring now to the almanac
of his skin tightening and happy
to not exercise fate
Newton's worm thinks,
why bother climbing
I can have it all
lying down.

Seed Kabbalist Tree

He saw her eyes holding
what was between them:
The apple bruised the skin
she'd bit; her mouth, record
of its bronze. New drift
of her lips light couldn't name.
He didn't know punishment.
How taste apple gender divide
word from rib all at once
Adamah, ground no water plants
whole again. When she ate
she became seed. He became
Kabbalist and tree.

Still Life

I

A pear
on a vendor's cart
reflects the granite slabbed Manhattan afternoon:
Tiger eyed stone climbs 100 storeys,
impales an invisible sky.
Yet as long as the bronze light lasts
the pear holds the street.
Taxis, doormen, vendors, even the men
manning pneumatic drills,
are arrested from their commercial sleep,
watching one pigeon flying across the noise
dying for the pear in the mirrored light.

The bronze gone,
the sweet juices spilled, the core
ground into pavement.

II

Under Brooklyn Bridge
skullbanger stone. Needles
drain the sun, veins balloon,
mainline delirium: Eye a gash of salt;
Ear a vice to put the squeeze on a shrill C note;
Trilled tongues roll from troughs like red carpets
to lick the blade, sport the gun.
A random bullet kills with such precision.

Hypodermic
the black orange of night
sucked dry.

III

Power of the eye that holds the pear
magnifies a thousand fold its size,
does not blur, blink or bless: The lubricant tear
washes the lids, steadies the sight: A welder's torch
illuminates the sky above Jewelry Row.

A silenced tongue
begs the knife
to slit the evening wide.

IV

The sleeping wound awakes.
Knock once, twice, the city, like a ganglion,
revives: Romulus drugged, Remus suckling fear.
Abscessed moon, the city is open for taking:
All the potted palms, all the artificial roses
in the lobby of love, rot. Outside in the benzine air
the borough's neck is taut: Jugular bulges,
Adam's Apple deftly exposed; Junkie Lazarus
rises through the cauterized throat.
The mouth opens. Its wind seared flesh
mutely blows.

A silenced tongue
begs the knife
to slit the evening wide.

Selections from *The Isaac Oratorio*

ERRATUM
p. 30, Section III should end

The satin held coin
pays for the diamond reins
dogging the city.

Sarah's Song

I was young once
could lose myself in the sand
moving across the desert night or
under the stars as you let down my hair
and we bedded till the ram's horn of sun
trumpeted morning. All this while Hagar lie awake
the light burning in her tent.
I remember the night you thought we conceived Isaac.
How could fire be so sweet and furious?
How could any moon not spill over its sides and rain
silver
on the pond in the oasis where we slept?
How we bathed that night and laughed.
So you'll understand if I ask how. Did I not put in
my days,
pound the stains out of lamb and fowl blood,
and earth stained cloth, rub the hides on flat stones,
shell the husks, and seed the fields for the bread I
made myself?
Is there something I didn't do or did poorly?
And yet I did all this in joy. We were a family.
If you couldn't forgive my sending Hagar away
I can only say in defense that I would have killed
for Isaac.
But you? What had you to lose? And what did you
expect?
I would greet you as if you were God's personal
surgeon,
severing light from the sun?

Are not the demands on this life enough without this
higher calling?
The only high calling is the owl in the tree who at
least sleeps
with an open eye. Not me. My nightmare is awake.
I can still see you licking the blade as you sharpen it
on the stone—the knife you used to kill our son. I can
imagine
that craggy hill with vultures like black sackcloth
decked on the trees
and you standing there with your sagging dry old
testicles
swinging like ruptured pendulums too old to tell
time.
Too old to make love to a woman but young enough
to kill a son?
And that last night when you told me you were tak-
ing him to school.
Maybe death is the best school to study afterlife.
No, a woman is faceless in your world.

*

Hagar's Complaint:

Hagar, haggard, hag, ragwoman me.
Tossed out, exiled, bought to supplant a barren womb.
I provided and was paid in kind, but you my son
denied.
Yes, promises were made, promises delayed,
but the promise of your father's God is born of
wandering.
I was a maid from the beginning: clean the master's
house,
iron his shirts (just so much starch), fix his eggs,
basted not poached, no poachers, no Ishmael to receive
his due as the true first son. So it's sweep the dust off
the floor and then "Sorry, Hagar, you're needed no
more."
What pleasures Abraham sought from me
he cheapened in not asking them of Sarah.
How many times did he spill his seed with her?
But our seed is exile. So I do not thank you, Sarah,
even though I am honored, even though I am the
beginning
of a holy line.

*

Sarah of the Double Laugh:

When God told me of this plan
I laughed again.
It was impossible to believe.
Was it a bet with the devil, a whim?
Was there a grievance with us
for God to break the bread of our trust?
So when I laughed twice
it must have seemed a double dare.
Did God wish to punish me
for seeming to know Abraham
would not touch a strand of Isaac's hair
and risk tearing the universe?
My faith was beyond Abraham
and Isaac was attached to that place in my womb
that bore God's face.

*

Chorus: "A Boy Has Died"

A boy has died.
Who will sing his song?
Who will play the violin for him?

A boy is gone.
Who will weep for him?

The leaves fall. The ground grows cold.
His soul won't rise
till someone weeps for him.

Will the windows remember his eyes?
Will the stairs he climbed rise up to heaven?
Will the streets run with him?
Will laughter follow his name?

A boy has died.
Who will weep for him?

*

The Sad Story of Isaac:

It is twenty years later. For Isaac the sacrifice has not faded like an old serigraph. Even after the years of electroshock therapy he remembers seeing everything and hearing everything except "Abraham, Abraham". The famous therapist told him he was blocked. But Isaac took exception. "You'll forgive the pun, Doctor," he said, "but my head was on the block."

Oddly, the sacrifice turned him into something of a lady's man, which he explains by saying when he retunred home and Sarah was dead he was inconsolable and ran off. Looking, looking, he's always looking for the understanding and mother love he lost when Sarah died. It's the same record with him. The same ritual he performs. He finds a sympathetic ear and tells his story. At the end of his tale he asks the woman of that night to remove the bandanna fastened around his neck. Some touch it. Some claim to feel the light of God in the scar. Others, the cold blade of Abraham. But they all make love to him, tenderly and passionately gripping his neck, trying to heal the heart under the wound. Isaac is happy for a moment but in the morning light the truth blares home and the woman leave never to return. That morning they discover callouses on their hands, scars that wail at noon.

*

Isaac Jerusalem Lion:

My neck is stretched out on the Eternal line.
Dawn binds my hands and legs.
Sunset shatters the last marrow of my hope.
I am Isaac of the wheat, of the chaff of the final hour.
My belly laugh covers the sorrow
of our mothers' hearts, the handiwork of our father's Gods,
I am Isaac, black letter of the law, red letter of the covenant.
Isaac of the phylactery joining yes and no.
Isaac who never shed a tear,
who lay still under his father's God-drugged eyes
who feels the stars' cool hands on my brow
and Paradise is the full moon's silver blood
gushing like a slain Jerusalem lion from my throat.

*

Afterword: Isaac at the Wailing Wall

Isaac, a little grumpy from the long hours on the bus, the overcooked meat, and the tour guide's deficient Hebrew, has seen all the sights, the marvels and inventions of the new world, the religions spawned. He's unimpressed with telecommunications and for him the elevator up to Masada promotes flab. After Golgotha and Yad Vashem he's feeling raw. "Who says no man crosses the same river twice," he tells, No One Listening. "All I see is the same bloody man crossing the same bloody river." He takes out a piece of paper and writes. "Take it all back," and stuffs it in a crack in the wall.

For an instant the black robes, the three cornered hats become raven cawing above; the white stones of the white streets fly into the wings of the dove; the red sea recedes into itself, and the mosque music from the four way speakers becomes the four pouring rivers out of Eden before dawn.

Isaac turns as he feels his father's heavy hand on his back, the long whiskers brushing his neck. He smells the stale Torah breath of a kosher, lawful God.

Abraham smiles. "There's nothing for us in this fortune cookie wall. Come, Isaac, it is time to go home."

*

About the Author

David Raffeld was born in South Chicago and has been a hod carrier, sheetrocker, painter, ballet manager and sculptor. A graduate of the University of Missouri at Columbia, he is the editor and publisher of *POTLATCXH* magazine. He is a frequent adjunct in the departments of Religion and Philosophy at Williams College, where he was also artist-in-residence during the production of his *The Isaac Oratorio* by the Theatre Department. His poems have appeared in *The Christian Science Monitor*, *Poetry East*, *Phoebe* and others. His first book, *The Ballad of Harmonica George & Other Poems*, was published by Adastra in 1989. He lives with his wife, Beth, son, Eli, and daughter, Miriam, in Williamstown, Massachusetts.

Colophon

Into the World of Men by David Raffeld is limited to 300 copies, 26 of which are cloth, signed and lettered A-Z by the author. Designed and printed letterpress from hand-set type then hand sewn by Gary Metras (with help from the author), December to January 96-97. Cloth copies hand-bound by David Bourbeau. Text paper is Classic Laid Natural with Genesis Rain for the cover; both are recycled and acid free. Type is Monotype Garamond Old Style, named for sixteenth century type designer Claude Garamond but actually designed by Jean Jannon, the seventeenth century Paris printer. Production labor was eased by the author's visits to the press and the ensuing good talk

* *
*